THE EMERGENCY ROOM:
WHEN DOES MY CHILD NEED TO GO?

How to manage common medical conditions that
affect children and when to call your doctor

by

Richard Greenberg, MD

TELEMACHUS PRESS

THE EMERGENCY ROOM: WHEN DOES MY CHILD NEED TO GO?

Cover designed by Carrie Greenberg and Telemachus Press, LLC

Author Photograph by Kristy Merrill

Nasal suction photograph of Jane Elizabeth Beck

Interior art:
Copyright © iStockphoto/34438450_FamVeld

Cover photograph of Marla Rae Greenberg

Published by Telemachus Press, LLC
http://www.telemachuspress.com

Visit the author's website:
http://www.ragbooks.com

ISBN: 978-1-939927-47-7 (eBook)
ISBN: 978-1-939927-48-4 (Paperback)

Version 2014.12.29

Second Edition

Printed in the United States of America

10 9 8 7 6 5 4 3 2 1

Disclaimer

All information, content, and material in this book is for informational purposes only and is not intended to serve as a substitute for the consultation, diagnosis, medical advice, and/or medical treatment of a medical illness or injury by a healthcare provider. If you suspect that your child has a serious condition, you should have him/her evaluated by a medical professional immediately.

Dedication

To my wife Carrie and my children Zachary, Samantha, and Marla, who support and inspire me. To my parents, Jack and Barbara, who gave me my love of medicine and taught me the importance of serving others. To my patients who continually motivate me to become a better doctor. To my family and friends who bring love to my life and to God who sustains me. Thank you.

Table of Contents

Introduction   i

1. Fever   1

2. Vomiting, Diarrhea, and Dehydration   8

3. Seizures   15

4. Coughs, Colds, and Sinus Infections   20

5. Ear Infections   26

6. Head Injuries   31

7. Bronchiolitis (and RSV)   36

8. Abdominal Pain and Constipation   41

9. Croup   45

10. Infections: Viruses versus Bacteria   49

11. Influenza   52

THE EMERGENCY ROOM:

WHEN DOES MY CHILD NEED TO GO?

How to manage common medical conditions that
affect children and when to call your doctor

Introduction

I am a pediatrician and pediatric emergency specialist. I am constantly caring for children in the middle of the night in the emergency room (ER). All too often they present to the ER with minor illnesses. When I take the time to thoroughly explain their child's condition, parents are very grateful. Many parents have expressed to me that having that information may have prevented a trip to the ER. Parents are often frustrated because they do not know when it is necessary to bring their child into the ER. As a father, I understand the concern that parents have when their children are ill. As a physician, I also understand the burden that parents have to endure waiting to be seen in the middle of the night.

The purpose of this book is to help parents understand more about common medical conditions that affect their children. I hope to give you the tools to understand when you need to be concerned enough to have your child evaluated by your doctor or be seen in the ER. Many children are brought to the ER because parents are concerned that their child may have a serious medical condition. As a pediatrician and pediatric ER doctor, I highly value the opinions and concerns of parents. However, oftentimes this high level of concern stems from some common misconceptions that I hope to address in this book.

An example of this scenario occurs when a child has a fever. Almost all parents believe that once a child's temperature reaches a certain number, the child needs to be evaluated immediately. I refer to this as "fever phobia." The concept that the height of a child's fever suggests a serious condition is simply not true (see *Chapter 1: Fever* for a full discussion). Parents should be educated properly regarding serious symptoms and their child's condition. Unfortunately, this type of education rarely happens sufficiently in the current busy medical environment. My purpose in writing this book is not to prevent you from visiting your doctor or the ER if you are a concerned parent. If a parent is truly concerned about his/her child, then it is best to have him/her evaluated immediately. I do hope to help you decide when to be concerned regarding your child's condition, so that you can make an informed decision regarding your child's need for medical care.

At the end of each chapter, I have listed key points to remember about each topic. In the key point section, I summarize the reasons that should prompt you to seek medical care for your child with your doctor or in an ER.

Chapter 1
Fever

Fever is the most common reason families bring their children to the emergency room. There is a lot of incorrect information regarding fever. What temperature, due to fever, is dangerous for my child? Will the fever cause brain damage? How often can I give fever medication? In this chapter, I will answer these and other common questions that parents often ask when in the ER.

Fever indicates that the body has some type of infection. It is the body's response to this infection. How do we define fever? Doctors consider a fever anything equal to or greater than 100.4°F. Fever is not dangerous to your child. I repeat: *Fever is not dangerous or harmful for your child.* In fact, many experts believe that fever is one of the mechanisms used by the body to fight infection. Many people have heard that fever can "fry the brain" or cause some type of brain damage. This common belief is simply not true. I have been asked countless times by parents, "What temperature is too high or dangerous for my child?" The answer often stuns parents: *There is no temperature that is too high or dangerous for a child.* I must comment here that there is no temperature that is dangerous for a child as long as the temperature is caused by fever. If a child is left in a car on a hot day and his/her temperature rises to a high level, the situation can be dangerous and even potentially deadly. A rise in body temperature due to fever, however, is the body's natural response to fight an infection and is not dangerous. Fever can be associated in some children with "fever seizures" (febrile seizures). See *Chapter 3: Seizures* for a discussion on this topic.

I want to clarify a point made earlier regarding fever. Fever indicates that a child has an infection. Some of these infections are mild and others can be serious. Although the fever itself is not dangerous, the infection that a child has might be dangerous. A good rule of thumb to know whether or not an infection is dangerous is to see how your child appears. I have told parents countless times that, as a doctor, I am more concerned with a child that appears ill with a fever of 101°F than a child that appears well and has a fever of 105°F. Just as adults feel and look lousy when they have a fever, so do children. When a child has a fever, it is okay for him/her to feel and look bad. However, when the child's fever is brought down and he/she continues to look poorly, then you should seek medical attention for your child. Children with very serious conditions, such as meningitis, do not look and act well when their fever resolves. Consider the analogy of a roller coaster. As a doctor, I expect that when a child has a fever, he/she will be cranky, will want to be held, and will not want to play. I also expect that as the fever comes down, the child may not be acting completely normally, but that he/she will improve and will want to be more active, less cranky, and will play. In the same way that a roller coaster has ups and downs, that is how a child's illness may often proceed. If a child continues to be fussy, ill-appearing, and/or does not improve with fever control measures, then that child should be seen by a doctor.

How should you treat your child's fever? There are two types of medications to treat fever: Ibuprofen (Motrin®, Advil®) and Acetaminophen (Tylenol®). Parents want to know how often they can use these medications to treat a fever. Many parents use a set alternating schedule of dosing medications every three or four hours around the clock to treat fever. I believe that this approach can be confusing for parents and may not be the best for the child.

Ibuprofen can be given every six to eight hours and Acetaminophen can be given every four to six hours. Most doctors do not recommend the use of Ibuprofen for children less than six months of age. If your child has a fever, choose one of the two medications, and ask yourself one simple question: Has it been at least X hours (six to eight hours or four to six hours, depending upon which medicine you will use) since the last dose? If you are using Ibuprofen to treat the fever then you only need to worry about when the last dose of Ibuprofen was given. If you are using Acetaminophen, then you only need to worry about when the last dose of Acetaminophen was given. The fact that seems to confuse parents is that it does not matter when the last dose of Ibuprofen was given relative to the last dose of Acetaminophen.

In fact, it would not hurt children to give them Ibuprofen and Acetaminophen at the same time as long as enough time has elapsed since their last dose of each medicine. I recommend treating a fever with one of the two medicines and waiting for an hour for that medicine to begin to work. If your child still has a fever, use the other of the two medicines, as long as it is time for that medication. Using this method, you do not need to wait another three or four hours to use another medicine for your child's fever. This method allows parents to tailor the treatment of fever to their child rather than using a set generic schedule. See the dosing charts at the end of this chapter.

You can also treat a fever by placing cool washcloths on your child's forehead and body. Also, lukewarm baths may be used to bring your child's temperature down. Children often feel cold ("the chills") when they have a fever. A parent's natural response is to cover the child with more clothes and blankets. Although this often comforts a child, it makes it harder to reduce the fever. I recommend that you minimize the amount of clothes/blankets used to help bring down the fever.

Parents often are concerned that the fever has not completely resolved with the use of the fever medicines. This is not concerning to me as a doctor. Remember that fever is not dangerous and simply indicates that your child has an infection. I will discuss types of infections later in the book. See *Chapter 10: Infections: Viruses versus Bacteria.*

When should you be concerned as a parent if your child has a fever? Children less than three months of age should be seen immediately (call your doctor or be seen in an emergency room for fever of 100.4°F or greater). If your child's fever lasts for five days then he/she should be evaluated by a doctor. If your child is lethargic, ill-appearing, does not improve with fever medicines, or has a stiff neck, then he/she should be evaluated by a doctor immediately. The word lethargic often means something different to parents than it does to doctors. Doctors define lethargic as a child that can barely be awakened, even with stimulation. Parents often define lethargic as less active than normal.

Key points to remember about Fever:

*Fever will not cause brain damage.

*There is no fever that is too high or dangerous.

*Fever is the body's response while fighting an infection.

*Treat the fever with Acetaminophen and/or Ibuprofen.

*Use cooling measures (baths or cool washcloths) to treat fever.

*__Reasons to see your doctor__: If your child's fever lasts for five days or your child does not appear better when the fever resolves.

*__Reasons to be seen in the ER__: If your child has a fever and is less than three months old, is lethargic, has a stiff neck, or is ill-appearing.

Acetaminophen Dosing Chart

Weight	Dosage (mg)	Infant's suspension 160 mg/5 ml	Children's suspension 160 mg/5 ml	Children's chewables 80 mg each	Jr. strength chewables 160 mg each
6-11 lbs	40	¼ tsp (1.25 ml)	¼ tsp (1.25 ml)		
12-17 lbs	80	½ tsp (2.5 ml)	½ tsp (2.5 ml)		
18-23 lbs	120	¾ tsp (3.75 ml)	¾ tsp (3.75 ml)		
24-35 lbs	160	1 tsp (5 ml)	1 tsp (5 ml)	2	
36-47 lbs	240	1 ½ tsp (7.5 ml)	1 ½ tsp (7.5 ml)	3	
48-59 lbs	320	2 tsp (10 ml)	2 tsp (10 ml)	4	2
60-71 lbs	400	2 ½ tsp (12.5 ml)	2 ½ tsp (12.5 ml)	5	2 ½
72-95 lbs	480	3 tsp (15 ml)	3 tsp (15 ml)	6	3
96+ lbs	640				4

Acetaminophen (Tylenol®) may be given every four to six hours.

Ibuprofen Dosing Chart

Weight	Dosage (mg)	Infant's drops 50mg/1.25 ml	Children's suspension 100 mg/5 ml	Chewable tablets 50 mg each	Chewable tablets 100 mg each
12-17 lbs	50	1 dropper (1.25 ml)	½ tsp (2.5 ml)		
18-23 lbs	75	1 ½ droppers (1.875 ml)	¾ tsp (3.75 ml)		
24-35 lbs	100	2 droppers (2.5 ml)	1 tsp (5 ml)	2	1
36-47 lbs	150		1 ½ tsp (7.5 ml)	3	1 ½
48-59 lbs	200		2 tsp (10 ml)	4	2
60-71 lbs	250		2 ½ tsp (12.5 ml)	5	2 ½
72-95 lbs	300		3 tsp (15 ml)	6	3
96+ lbs	400		4 tsp (20 ml)	8	4

Ibuprofen (Motrin®, Advil®) may be given every six to eight hours. Do not use Ibuprofen until a child reaches six months of age.

Chapter 2
Vomiting, Diarrhea, and Dehydration

Vomiting and/or diarrhea are common reasons for children to present to the emergency room. The most common cause of vomiting and diarrhea is gastroenteritis, which refers to inflammation/infection in the intestinal tract. This condition is caused by different viruses. One of the most common viruses causing gastroenteritis is Rotavirus. However, there are several other common viruses that cause this condition. There is no cure for any of the viruses associated with gastro-enteritis. However, there is a vaccine that can help prevent gastroenteritis caused by Rotavirus. Symptoms from this illness can last from less than one day to one week depending upon the child and the severity of illness.

The most common concern that parents have with these symptoms is that their child is dehydrated. Dehydration is the most common complication associated with gastroenteritis. How do you know if your child is dehydrated? Children that are dehydrated often have dry lips/mouth, sunken eyes, and are more sleepy/less active. Children often will have a significant decrease in the amount of urine made when they are dehydrated. If a young child has diarrhea, however, it can be difficult to tell how much urine they are having as it is often mixed in with the diarrhea in the diaper. See Figure 1 for an illustration of the signs of dehydration.

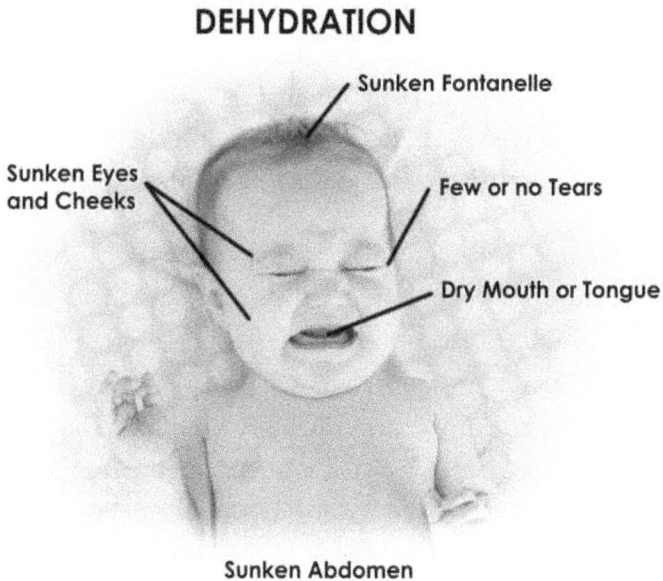

DEHYDRATION

Sunken Fontanelle

Sunken Eyes and Cheeks

Few or no Tears

Dry Mouth or Tongue

Sunken Abdomen

Figure 1. Signs of Dehydration in a Child

What can you do to help your child? Give your child small amounts of clear liquids frequently. The best choice is an electrolyte solution (Pedialyte® or other generic brands). I prefer the generic store brand as it contains the same basic ingredients and often costs much less. If your child will not take an electrolyte solution, then the next best thing to use is a Gatorade® type drink. The stomach becomes very irritated with this illness and can often handle only very small amounts at a time. Sometimes children can only handle one teaspoon (five ml) of liquid at a time. I recommend using a syringe of five ml every five to ten minutes. When your child can tolerate this without vomiting then increase the amount you give each time very slowly. When your child can tolerate a normal amount of liquid at one time (this will vary from three to eight ounces depending upon the child's age), then and only then should you try giving him/her something other than clear liquids (Pedialyte® or Gatorade® type drinks).

Popsicles are also good to give to children. These are effective because they are considered a clear liquid and children usually cannot eat them too quickly. Children often will want to take more than the small amount recommended. It can be difficult as a parent to deny your sick child more liquids and make him/her wait five to ten minutes for the next round. I often see parents give in to their children's crying, and this unfortunately leads to an increased risk of vomiting. I understand as a parent the difficulty in making your child wait a few more minutes for that next sip, but that may be what is best for him/her.

Once your child can tolerate several ounces at a time consistently without vomiting, then it is time to advance the diet. I recommend using easy foods and avoiding milk until they can tolerate other solids. Milk, although a kid favorite, is very hard on the stomach and can induce vomiting. I recommend using the BRAT diet, which consists of bananas, rice, applesauce, and toast. Try small amounts of these foods at a time. Once your child can consistently hold down these foods, then it is safe to try milk. If at any time your child starts to vomit again then move back to the previous step in the hydration chain (clear liquids → BRAT foods → milk and other foods).

It is best to avoid giving your child water. This is confusing to parents because, as adults, we often prefer water to help our dehydration. The difference with children is that their kidneys are not as advanced as adult kidneys. When children have vomiting and diarrhea, they lose fluids (water) and electrolytes (blood salts such as sodium and potassium). If you replace just water, then it can dilute the existing electrolytes in a child's bloodstream, which can be dangerous. If given enough water, a child's sodium level can decrease, which can cause seizures.

Parents are concerned with the fact that, for days, their child is only taking liquids and not solids when following the above outlined strategy. It is okay for children to live on liquids only and not to have solids for several days. When a child is sick, I tell parents to forget everything that pediatricians preach regarding taking in enough calories to sustain growth and development. When a child is ill, the main concern is maintaining good hydration.

Does my child need an intravenous line (IV) for fluids? This is the most common reason that children are brought to the ER. Most children do not require an IV for gastroenteritis. Children with moderate to severe dehydration will require IV fluids. Children with mild to moderate dehydration can often be treated with small sips of clear liquids. If they tolerate this regimen then IV fluids are not needed. If they continue to vomit, then IV fluids may be needed. Children with mild dehydration do not need IV fluids. Remember: There is no cure for this illness and once you have been seen by your doctor, your child will likely have more vomiting and/or diarrhea. Your goal is to get more in than comes out. This can often be difficult to know. I recommend that you use the signs of dehydration (see Figure 1) mentioned earlier as a guide to determine if your child needs medical attention.

Should my child receive anti-nausea medicine? Most anti-nausea medicines are dangerous for children. Despite this fact, many doctors still prescribe them to children. The FDA banned the use of one of the most common anti-nausea medicines, Phenergan® (generic name Promethazine), in children under the age of two years because of the risk of breathing difficulties and death. Many of the anti-nausea medicines have common and serious side effects in children. One of the newer anti-nausea medicines, Zofran® (generic name Ondansetron), has very few side effects in children. I believe that Zofran® is safe to use in children that require an anti-nausea medicine.

Should my child receive anti-diarrheal medicine? Most anti-diarrheal medicines can have significant side effects for children. Even those medicines labeled as pediatric or for kids can be dangerous. For instance, Pepto-Bismol® and Kaopectate® contain bismuth subsalicylate, which is an aspirin-like compound. Aspirin can be dangerous for children. Medication such as Immodium® can also be dangerous for children. The only safe anti-diarrheal medication that I recommend is probiotics. This type of medication is designed to add "good" bacteria back into the intestines because diarrhea causes an imbalance of bacteria. Probiotics can be found over the counter at most stores.

When should I be concerned if my child has vomiting or diarrhea? With gastroenteritis, children will often start vomiting first and then later develop diarrhea. Younger children almost always have both symptoms whereas older children may only vomit with minimal to no diarrhea. If a child is only vomiting, then other conditions can be the cause. Gastroenteritis can cause a child to have a fever. However, urinary tract infections can also cause fever, vomiting, and sometimes diarrhea. If your child is a girl under three years, or a boy under one year and has persistent fever associated with vomiting/diarrhea, then you should consider having him/her checked for a urinary infection. Crampy abdominal pain is common in gastroenteritis. The abdominal pain often occurs right before or after the child has started vomiting and/or has diarrhea.

If your child has worsening abdominal pain, consistent abdominal pain, or abdominal pain on their right side, then you should call or see a doctor immediately to evaluate for appendicitis or other serious conditions. Also, if your child has blood in the vomit or stool, or has all green vomit (bile), then you should see a doctor. Parents often confuse the yellow stomach acid as bile. Bile is a "pea soup" green and is produced further down the gastrointestinal tract than the stomach. Bile in the vomit can suggest a blockage in the intestines, which can be very serious. Sometimes children will vomit small amounts of green mucous and this is not concerning. When a child vomits bile, the entire vomit will be green. If it is mucous, then there will be chunks of green mucous within the vomit that is clear or yellow.

The symptoms of gastroenteritis should be gone in one week. Although I have seen them persist longer, if they do last longer than seven days, you should see a doctor for an evaluation. If the diarrhea lasts for greater than seven days, then your doctor should consider sending stool samples to check for bacterial infections, Giardia, and other conditions.

Key points to remember about
Vomiting, Diarrhea, and Dehydration:

*Most commonly caused by a virus and there is no cure.

*Offer small amounts of clear liquids frequently.

*Watch for the signs of dehydration (sunken eyes, dry lips/mouth, and sleepiness).

*Watch for bile (green) or blood in vomit, blood in stool, or worsening abdominal pain.

***Reasons to see your doctor**: If there are signs of dehydration or blood in the vomit or stool.

***Reasons to be seen in the ER**: If your child vomits bile (green), appears severely dehydrated, or has worsening abdominal pain.

Chapter 3
Seizures

Seizures are a common condition in children. A seizure is abnormal and uncontrolled electrical brain activity that leads to physical convulsions. The most common variety of seizure in children is called a tonic-clonic seizure, also known as a grand mal seizure. With a tonic-clonic seizure, children will have stiffening and jerking episodes that are repetitive and usually involve both arms and legs. It is common during a seizure for a child's eyes to have abnormal movements and also for them to have stool and urinary accidents. After a seizure is finished, a child will typically be sleepy (known as the postictal period) for at least 10-15 minutes or longer. There are other types of seizures such as staring spells (absence seizures), seizures associated with fever (febrile seizures), and multiple other types. Epilepsy is a seizure disorder in which patients have multiple seizures throughout their lifetime. Although seizures are a scary event for the family, they are rarely harmful to the child. A seizure will not "fry the brain" or cause brain damage as long as it does not last longer than 10-15 minutes and the child is maintaining a good oxygen level (not turning blue).

Seizures associated with fever (febrile seizures or fever seizures) are very common. Approximately five percent of children ages six months to six years will have a febrile seizure. There is no way to predict or prevent your child from having a febrile seizure. This type of seizure is caused by a child's fever rapidly spiking. The most common type of febrile seizure is a full body tonic-clonic seizure as described in the above paragraph. Typically, febrile seizures last less than 15 minutes. Your child will be sleepy and difficult to arouse after the seizure stops. I will discuss what to do if your child has a seizure later in this chapter. Once your child's seizure has stopped, you should call your doctor or have your child evaluated in an emergency room. If your child returns to normal after the sleepy period of the seizure, then doctors will typically not perform any testing to evaluate the seizure. Doctors may need to perform some evaluation to determine the cause of your child's fever. The majority (up to 99 percent) of children with febrile seizures will not go on to have epilepsy (a seizure disorder). However, children that have a febrile seizure are at increased risk to have further febrile seizures until they reach the age of six years. As a parent of a child that had a febrile seizure, I share in the concern that parents have regarding the possibility of further seizures. If your child develops a fever, treat him/her with fever medicines and lukewarm baths (see *Chapter 1: Fever*). Treatment with these measures has been shown not to prevent further seizures, but will often make children and their parents feel better.

Any child having a non-fever induced seizure will require an evaluation for that seizure. This may involve some type of x-ray of the brain such as an MRI or a CT (CAT) scan. Also, an electroencephalogram (EEG), an electrical brain wave test, will typically be performed to evaluate for abnormal brain wave activity that may lead to a seizure. Blood tests, which will check electrolytes (blood salts, such as sodium, potassium, calcium, and glucose) are typically run. An electrocardiogram (EKG), an electrical heart rhythm test, is also frequently performed. Once your child's seizure is over, you should call your doctor or have your child evaluated in an emergency room. In the ER, if a child has returned to normal, it is common to perform blood tests to check the electrolytes and to refer the child to a seizure specialist (a neurologist) to determine if an EEG and x-rays are needed. Also, the specialist will determine if treatment with anti-seizure medicines is needed.

What should you do if your child has a seizure? First of all, forget everything you have ever seen on TV shows. If your child starts to have a seizure, place him/her in a safe place to have the seizure. If he/she is on a bed or couch, then lay him/her on the floor so he/she will not fall during the seizure. Place your child on his/her side in case there is vomiting. This will help prevent the child from aspirating (inhaling into the lungs) if there is vomiting. Do not put your hand in your child's mouth to manipulate the tongue. As long as your child is breathing (watch the chest for up and down movement) and not turning blue in the face, allow your child to have a seizure for up to five minutes. It is best to look at a watch or clock because five minutes of watching your child have a seizure will seem like an eternity. You do not need to call **911** unless your child is not breathing, is turning blue, or if the seizure lasts longer than five minutes. Once the seizure has stopped, call your doctor or have your child seen in the ER.

A child that has had a seizure needs to be watched more closely in certain aspects of his/her life (seizure precautions). Essentially parents need to think of potentially dangerous situations that may arise if a child has a seizure. For instance, if your child is old enough to take a bath on his or her own, it would be dangerous if he/she had a seizure during the bath. Therefore, it would be better for him/her to take a shower and have someone listen to him/her in the shower to make sure that a seizure has not taken place. Also, if a child was climbing a tree and had a seizure, this could pose a significant risk. Finally, your child needs to be monitored very closely while swimming. I recommend that any child with a history of seizures have an adult assigned to specifically watch that child during swimming. That adult should not be watching other children at the same time.

Key points to remember about Seizures:

*Seizures are common in children, especially febrile seizures.

*If your child has a seizure, place him/her in a safe place, lay the child on his or her side, and do not put your finger (or anything else) in the child's mouth.

***Reasons to see your doctor**: For evaluation after your child has a seizure (as long as your child returns to baseline after the post seizure period).

***Reasons to be seen in the ER**: If your child does not return to normal after the seizure.

***Reasons to call 911**: If your child stops breathing, turns blue, or has a seizure lasting longer than five minutes.

Chapter 4
Coughs, Colds, and Sinus Infections

Respiratory symptoms are one of the most common reasons that parents bring their children to see a doctor. These symptoms are very common, especially during wintertime. The majority of these infections are caused by viruses (see *Chapter 10: Infections: Viruses versus Bacteria*). Symptoms of typical viral respiratory infections are nasal congestion, runny nose, cough, and fever. In addition, children often do not want to eat during the illness. Physicians will tell parents that infections from viruses only last five to seven days. Although this statement is true in many instances, it may not be true for respiratory viruses. Children can have a runny nose for a few weeks with respiratory viral infections. Also, once the infection has run its course, a cough can persist for a few more weeks due to irritation in the respiratory tract from the viral infection. It is not common for the fever to last for more than five days with these types of viral infections.

One of the most common misconceptions among parents and doctors is that once a child has a runny nose for more than ten days, then it must be a sinus infection (sinusitis) and requires antibiotics. This is simply not true. A sinus infection is a bacterial infection that requires antibiotics. Children are born with only a small percentage of their sinuses already developed. It takes several years for the full development of the sinuses to take place. Sinusitis is one of the most commonly over-diagnosed and misdiagnosed conditions in children. As parents, we all want to do something to help our children when they are sick. This is one compelling factor that leads parents to ask doctors to prescribe antibiotics for their children. Many doctors would rather give in to parents' demands than stand up for what is right for children and for the practice of good medicine. Unfortunately, the improper use of antibiotics can be very harmful for individual children and the community as well, due to the development of antibiotic resistance. I will discuss the concept of resistance to antibiotics later in the book. See *Chapter 10: Infections: Viruses versus Bacteria.*

Bacterial sinusitis is very uncommon in children. Typical symptoms of this condition include persistent fevers, headache, facial pain, as well as nasal congestion and runny nose that last longer than 10 days. If your child is experiencing these symptoms, a course of antibiotics may be required. Also, the color of the nasal drainage does not predict whether it is caused by a virus or by bacteria. Viral infections often produce green or yellow nasal drainage. The color change simply implies that white blood cells, one of the body's defense mechanisms, have come to fight the infection.

Coughs and colds are almost always caused by viruses. Antibiotics will not help cure infections caused by viruses. In the ER, parents often state that the last time their child had respiratory symptoms he/she received a course of antibiotics and that his/her symptoms got better within a few days. My response to them is that their child's symptoms would have likely resolved on their own within that same time frame if antibiotics had not been prescribed. Although I use antibiotics frequently as a physician, I strongly believe that the misuse and abuse of antibiotics in children has led to our current problem of antibiotic resistance. Please remember, as parents, that pressuring your doctor to prescribe antibiotics to your child may hurt him/her in the future.

Another potential complication of a cold is pneumonia. Pneumonia implies that there is a bacterial infection of the lungs. Only a small percentage of children with cough and cold symptoms develop pneumonia. A chest x-ray should be obtained to diagnose pneumonia. Children with pneumonia often have high fever, look ill, and breathe very fast. In general, children often breathe fast when they have a high fever, but this resolves when the fever is brought down. Children with pneumonia often breathe fast even when they do not have a fever. Children with simple colds can have similar symptoms to children with pneumonia and, therefore, your doctor needs to determine if a chest x-ray is needed.

Infants can benefit from nasal suction when they have significant congestion. I recommend using saline (salt water) with the nasal suction to loosen the mucous. Place a few drops of the saline in each nostril. Compress one nostril while using the bulb syringe to suck out the other nostril (See Figure 2). Repeat the process on the other side. Many parents believe that humidifiers help children with respiratory illnesses. Although research studies have not shown a significant difference with the use of humidifiers, I believe that it is a simple measure that is worthwhile. Cough and cold medicines generally DO NOT WORK in children. Multiple research studies, as well as countless reports from parents, confirm this fact. I do not recommend the use of these medicines for children with colds. Although as parents we want to do something to help our children, using these medicines has almost no chance of benefit and actually can have significant risks. Recent reports have shown that even over-the-counter cough and cold medicines can be harmful or even deadly for very young children.

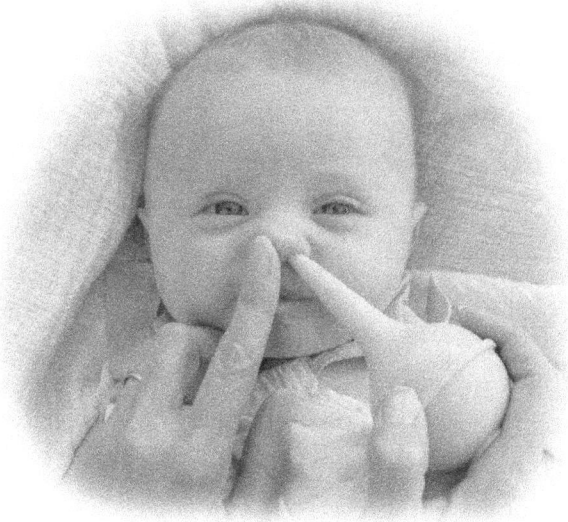

Figure 2. Proper Technique of Nasal Suction

Children often will not eat well when they are sick, especially with respiratory symptoms. It is more important to make sure that your child stays hydrated by drinking plenty of fluids than to be concerned regarding how much food they are eating. Please see *Chapter 2: Vomiting, Diarrhea, and Dehydration* for a discussion on the signs of dehydration.

When should you be concerned enough to have your child with respiratory symptoms evaluated by a doctor? You should have your child seen by a doctor if he/she is breathing fast, breathing hard (pulling in of the muscles near the ribs), or looks dehydrated. If your child has severe respiratory distress or turns blue, your child needs to be evaluated in the ER immediately. Call **911** if your child stops breathing, turns blue, or has severe respiratory distress. If your child's fever has lasted for five days, he/she should be seen by your doctor for an evaluation.

Key points to remember about
Coughs, Colds, and Sinus infections:

*Coughs and colds are almost always caused by viruses and there is no cure for them.

*Sinus infections are very uncommon in children.

*Antibiotics are rarely indicated for children with respiratory symptoms.

*Avoid cough and cold medicines unless directed otherwise by your doctor.

***Reasons to see your doctor**: If your child is breathing hard or fast, looks dehydrated, or if his/her fever lasts for five days.

***Reasons to be seen in the ER**: For severe respiratory distress, turning blue, stopping breathing, or lethargy.

Chapter 5
Ear Infections

Ear infections are a common condition in childhood. They are often associated with a cold. The cold causes swelling (inflammation) that interferes with drainage from the ear tubes (Eustachian tubes). This lack of drainage causes fluid to remain for a longer time in the middle ear (behind the ear drum). This stagnant fluid is a perfect breeding ground for bacteria, which can lead to an ear infection. Although ear infections are relatively common, they are probably one of the most over-diagnosed conditions in childhood.

There are two types of ear infections. A middle ear infection (otitis media) is the most common type of ear infection (described in the first paragraph). This type of infection can be caused by a virus or by bacteria. This will need to be determined by your doctor. If it is caused by bacteria, antibiotics will be needed. If it is caused by a virus, antibiotics will not help (see *Chapter 10: Infections: Viruses versus Bacteria*).

The second type of ear infection, an infection of the ear canal (otitis externa), is also known as swimmer's ear. This type of infection can happen with no exposure to swimming. This infection is caused by bacteria and should be treated with antibiotic drops to be placed in the ear. Children with swimmer's ear will often have a lot of pain when the outside of the ear is touched. Children with middle ear infections have ear pain, but this is not worsened by movement of the outside of the ear. For the purposes of the rest of this chapter, when I refer to ear infections, I will only be discussing middle ear infections.

Typical symptoms of ear infections are ear pain, ear pressure, pulling at ears, fussiness, not sleeping well, and poor feeding. Please note: I left out high fever as a symptom of ear infections. I know this may shock you, but ear infections do not cause high fever. As I mentioned earlier, ear infections are most commonly associated with colds. Colds are viral infections that can cause fever. Therefore, when a child has a cold and then gets an ear infection, he/she may get a fever. This fever is caused by the cold and not the ear infection. I have treated many children that have had ear infections that have never developed a fever. This may seem unimportant to you as a parent regarding whether or not ear infections truly cause a fever, but I believe it is very important for you to understand.

As an emergency room physician for children, I have seen hundreds of cases where a child's fever was incorrectly blamed on an ear infection. Unfortunately, in some of these cases, the fever was caused by serious infections such as meningitis and urinary tract infections. Many practitioners will diagnose an ear infection because it is common, and parents will be satisfied because a diagnosis has been made and an antibiotic prescription will be given. If your child has a high fever, it may be caused by the cold or it may be caused by other more serious infections, and you should discuss this with your doctor. If your child is less than one month of age, it is not appropriate for your child to be diagnosed with an ear infection without first having an evaluation for more serious conditions. This young age is when it is most likely that ear infections are misdiagnosed instead of meningitis. Although it is common for children to be fussy with ear infections, it is not common for them to be inconsolable. If you cannot do anything to calm and soothe your child's crying, other serious conditions should be considered.

When your young child pulls on his/her ear(s), it may be developmental as they are learning to explore their body, or it may be due to pain. The only way to know is to have your doctor check your baby's ears. When your child complains of ear pain and the doctor tells you that the ears appear normal, this is likely because your child is experiencing ear pressure. This pressure is due to the build-up of fluid in the middle ear caused by poor drainage due to a cold, as described earlier in this chapter. This pressure can cause pain, and the fluid sitting there can lead to an ear infection. It is common for a child's ears to look normal one day and then look infected a day or two later. Therefore, if your doctor tells you that the ears look normal and then a day or two later your child's pain or symptoms worsen, it is appropriate to have your child rechecked. It is not appropriate to just start antibiotics if your child has pain but the ears appear normal (see *Chapter 4: Cough, Colds, and Sinus Infections*).

Your doctor will discuss what type of antibiotic is appropriate to treat an ear infection. As more research is done, doctors are being more aggressive about just observing children with milder ear infections without using antibiotics. The trend toward using fewer antibiotics may help steer us away from developing antibiotic resistance. See *Chapter 4: Cough, Colds, and Sinus Infections* and *Chapter10: Infections: Viruses versus Bacteria*. Ear tubes are not required for most children. However, if children have repeated ear infections or do not improve on standard antibiotic regimens, then ear tubes may need to be placed. This should be determined by having a discussion with your doctor.

Rare complications of ear infections include meningitis and mastoiditis. Meningitis is a serious infection of the membrane layers that cover the brain and spinal cord. Children with this condition are inconsolable and have a stiff neck. Mastoiditis is a condition where the ear infection has spread to the bony air space behind the ear. This causes swelling behind the ear such that the ear sticks out away from the head. If your child is inconsolable to soothing measures, has a stiff neck, or has swelling behind the ear that causes the ear to protrude, you should have your child seen in the ER.

Key points to remember about Ear Infections:

*Ear infections do not cause high fever.

*If your child is less than one month of age or is difficult to console, consider more serious causes of fever (such as meningitis).

*Discuss with your doctor if antibiotics are truly needed in your child's case.

***Reasons to see your doctor**: If you are concerned your child has an ear infection.

***Reasons to be seen in the ER**: If your child is difficult to console, has a stiff neck, or swelling behind the ear.

Chapter 6
Head Injuries

Head injuries are one of the most common reasons that parents bring their children to the ER for evaluation. Most head injuries are relatively minor. However, a small percentage of head injuries are life threatening. As a parent, it is important to know the indications for having your child evaluated on an emergency basis.

Many children cry vigorously after hitting their head. It is common for children to fall asleep after this crying episode. Many parents believe that if their child falls asleep after the head trauma that the child may never wake up. This notion is only true in melodramatic television shows. Children that fall asleep after crying appropriately from their head trauma are usually falling asleep because they tire themselves out from crying or are in need of a nap. This is very different from a child who is excessively sleepy or one who cannot be aroused after hitting his/her head. This latter situation is concerning for serious head trauma. If your child hits his/her head and then cries and acts appropriately, it is okay to let your child fall asleep. If you feel comfortable that he or she is sleeping because he/she is tired, then just monitor your child at home. After an appropriate amount of nap time, wake your child up to see how he/she is doing. If your child does not act appropriately after head trauma or seems excessively sleepy, you should have your child evaluated in an emergency room.

Children can display several symptoms after experiencing head trauma. Vomiting is one of these common symptoms. Most children who vomit after head trauma have experienced a concussion (see discussion regarding concussion later in the chapter). Children who have a few isolated episodes of vomiting, but are otherwise acting normally, may be monitored at home. Children that have repetitive or persistent vomiting should be evaluated in the ER for serious head trauma.

Dizziness is another common symptom that indicates a concussion. If your child is dizzy but otherwise acting appropriately, it is okay to monitor him/her at home. Headaches are also possible after head trauma. If your child has a mild headache after hitting his/her head, it is appropriate to use Ibuprofen and/or Acetaminophen and monitor your child at home. If the headache is severe or persists after trying medication, then you should have your child evaluated in the ER. Seizures are an uncommon but possible symptom after head trauma. If your child has a seizure after hitting his/her head, he/she should be evaluated in an ER.

A concussion indicates that your child's brain has sustained an injury. Typical symptoms of a concussion are headache, vomiting, dizziness, blurred vision, and memory loss. Children that lose consciousness after head trauma, by definition, have experienced a concussion. Symptoms from a concussion can last from hours to several weeks and can range from mild to severe. The recommended treatment for a concussion is rest and good hydration. It is possible to have future learning deficits after experiencing a concussion. Some experts believe that your child might benefit from a few days of mental as well as physical rest after experiencing a significant concussion. You may consider having your child stay home from school for a few days if he/she is experiencing significant symptoms.

It is very important to have your child refrain from any contact sports or significant physical activity to prevent another concussion. If your child experiences a concussion, he/she should avoid contact sports for at least one to two weeks after returning to their normal state. This means that you should wait until your child has no concussion symptoms (no headache, memory problems, dizziness, etc.) and remains without symptoms for one to two weeks before allowing him/her to return to play. Your child should receive a medical screening exam by his/her physician prior to returning to sports. In addition, most experts agree that repetitive concussions will lead to learning disabilities and can even lead to death.

The injury to the brain in a concussion is not visible on a CT (CAT) scan or an MRI. If your child exhibits typical concussion symptoms after head trauma it is okay to observe him or her at home. As mentioned earlier, if your child has persistent or severe headache, persistent vomiting, or excessive sleepiness, then he/she should be evaluated in an ER.

Many children will get a "goose-egg" on their head after head trauma. Young children (0-18 months) that have this bump are at increased risk for a skull fracture or bleeding in the brain and should be evaluated in an ER. Children older than 18 months who have a bump of this sort can usually be observed at home. If the bump is extremely tender to the touch or your child is not acting appropriately, then call your doctor or have your child evaluated in the ER.

Many parents bring their child to the ER to get a CT scan to evaluate for significant head trauma. You should be aware of the risks and benefits of a CT scan. A CT scan is a great test to look for head trauma. It is very good at detecting skull fractures and bleeding in the head. A CT scan is not without risk, however. A CT scan will give your child a large dose of radiation. This radiation will not harm your child today or tomorrow, but does increase the risk of having cancer in the future. Therefore, you should discuss with your doctor if a CT scan is truly needed.

Key points to remember about Head Injuries:

*Discuss the benefits and risks of a CT scan with your doctor.

*Reasons to see your doctor: If your child is less than 18 months of age and has a "goose-egg," or if you are uncomfortable observing your child at home.

*Reasons to be seen in the ER: Your child has severe/persistent headache, is excessively sleepy, has persistent vomiting, or had a seizure associated with the head trauma.

Chapter 7
Bronchiolitis (and RSV)

Bronchiolitis is a common respiratory condition that occurs mainly during winter. This illness causes mucous production and inflammation in the lower respiratory airways. Although some people have not heard of bronchiolitis, most people have heard of RSV, which stands for Respiratory Syncytial Virus. This virus is the most common cause of bronchiolitis and is often synonymous with the illness. RSV is only one of many viruses that can cause bronchiolitis. The majority of children with this illness will have a very bad upper respiratory illness, i.e., a bad cold. The illness typically lasts about a week, but symptoms can linger for up to two weeks. Occasionally, this illness can cause severe respiratory symptoms requiring children to be placed on a ventilator (respirator). The severe manifestation of this disease is most common among children that are young (less than six months) and especially among infants who were born prematurely.

As a respiratory illness, the most common symptoms associated with bronchiolitis are cough, congestion, runny nose, fever, and poor feeding. Children will commonly get wheezing associated with this illness as well. Unfortunately, these symptoms seem to peak during the night, and it is common for children to sleep poorly. The mucous production and inflammation in the airways combined with the congestion cause children to have difficulty breathing. This can be manifested by nasal flaring (nose flares out when breaths are taken) and retractions (children use the muscles below and between the rib cage to take in breaths causing a "sucking-in" appearance in those locations). There is a significant range in the severity of illness with bronchiolitis. As mentioned earlier, most children simply have a really bad cold. A small percentage of children with a more significant illness will require hospitalization.

There is no specific treatment or cure for this illness. As a virus (see *Chapter 10: Infections: Viruses versus Bacteria*), the infection will need time to run its course and will resolve without treatment. This is a very difficult concept for parents because it is hard to accept that there is no specific treatment for this illness while their children are miserable with these symptoms. This illness is very different from bronchitis. Bronchitis is a condition that is similar to bronchiolitis, but it only occurs in adults. Physicians will often prescribe antibiotics for bronchitis, but antibiotics will not help in bronchiolitis. Although there is no cure for bronchiolitis, it can be spread easily from person to person. The illness is spread from respiratory secretions. The best way to prevent the spread of this illness is to avoid contact with other children that are ill with respiratory symptoms, cover children's mouths and noses when they cough/sneeze, and wash hands (yours and your child's hands) frequently.

There are some measures of supportive care, which can help lessen the severity of the symptoms. Suctioning the nose can help alleviate some of the nasal congestion. It is best to place some saline (salt water) up each nostril before suctioning the nose. Use of the saline will help loosen the mucous and make it easier to suction. You can purchase saline nasal wash at the store or you can make your own by mixing one-quarter teaspoon of salt with eight ounces of warm water. Place a few drops of saline in each nostril and then press on the right nostril while suctioning the left side, then repeat on the other side. See Figure 2 in *Chapter 4: Coughs, Colds, and Sinus Infections*. Many parents believe that using humidifiers helps children with respiratory illnesses. Although research studies have not shown a significant difference with the use of humidifiers, I believe that it is a simple measure and is worth trying.

Hydration is another major issue with this illness. It is difficult for children to eat and drink sufficiently with the significant congestion associated with bronchiolitis. Nasal suctioning can help with this. It is most important to encourage the taking of liquids over foods. Watch for the signs of dehydration (see *Chapter 2: Vomiting, Diarrhea and Dehydration*). The use of a nebulizer treatment with Albuterol (a respiratory medication used to treat asthma) will help a small percentage of children that have wheezing associated with this condition. There is an injection that can help prevent RSV in infants.

This is a very expensive medicine, and it is only used for children who were born prematurely or who have significant health issues such as heart disease. (See your doctor for guidelines regarding the use of this medicine).

Only a small percentage of children with this illness will require hospitalization. The reasons for hospitalization include respiratory distress, low oxygen level, or dehydration. If a child exhibits signs of significant respiratory distress (retractions, nasal flaring, and breathing fast) he/she may need to be admitted to the hospital for observation. It is important to monitor children for signs of worsening respiratory distress. Children that have severe distress may require the use of a ventilator to help them breathe. There is no way for you to tell that your child has a low oxygen level unless the level is severely low and your child is turning blue. In your doctor's office and in hospitals there are machines that can check a child's oxygen level with the use of a special "band-aid" appearing device placed on your child's hand or foot. If the oxygen level is low, your child may need to be hospitalized to receive oxygen. Finally, some children with bronchiolitis have such significant congestion that they are unable to keep sufficiently hydrated. When this happens, children may require hospitalization for IV fluid hydration.

If your child appears dehydrated or is breathing fast, you should call your doctor or be seen in the ER. If your child has significant respiratory distress, turns blue, or is lethargic (see definition of lethargic in *Chapter 1: Fever*), your child should be evaluated in the ER immediately.

Key points to remember about Bronchiolitis (and RSV):

*Monitor for signs of respiratory distress (nasal flaring, retractions, turning blue, and breathing fast).

*Monitor for signs of dehydration (sunken eyes, dry lips/mouth, and sleepiness).

*Bulb-suction the nose with saline to help with congestion.

*Have patience: This is a frustrating illness for parents as it will last for about a week or longer, and there is no cure to help your miserable child.

***Reasons to see your doctor**: If your child appears dehydrated or is breathing fast.

***Reasons to be seen in the ER**: If your child has significant respiratory distress, turns blue, or is lethargic.

Chapter 8
Abdominal Pain and Constipation

Abdominal pain is another common reason that brings parents into the ER. There are many causes of abdominal pain; most are not serious. One of the most common causes of abdominal pain in children is constipation. In this chapter, I will discuss how to distinguish serious causes of abdominal pain (e.g. appendicitis) from less serious causes.

When a child develops abdominal pain, parents often fear that their child has appendicitis. Children with appendicitis usually develop a mild aching pain around their belly button. This pain gradually worsens and moves to the right lower side of the abdomen. The pain with appendicitis is usually constant and does not come and go as with many other conditions. Children with appendicitis often have a low-grade fever, nausea/vomiting, and a poor appetite. Not all children with appendicitis develop these associated symptoms. There are definitely cases of appendicitis that do not follow the usual course of symptoms. This unusual course of symptoms typically happens in the very young patients (less than four years old). Young patients with appendicitis may have pain that comes and goes rather than the typical constant pain. If you suspect that your child has appendicitis, you should have him/her evaluated that day by your doctor or seen in the ER.

There are many different types of infections that manifest themselves with abdominal pain. Urinary tract infections often cause lower mid-abdominal pain. These patients often have pain with urination, fever, and vomiting. Pneumonia is another cause of abdominal pain. Children with pneumonia typically have fever, cough, and a rapid breathing rate. Throat infections (sore throat) can also be associated with abdominal pain. Strep throat is well known to be associated with abdominal pain. The abdominal pain with a sore throat typically comes and goes and is less severe than that of appendicitis. Another infection that is commonly associated with abdominal pain is gastroenteritis—a virus that causes vomiting and diarrhea (see *Chapter 2: Vomiting, Diarrhea, and Dehydration*). The pain with this condition also typically comes and goes and is often diffuse over the entire abdomen.

Constipation is the most common cause of abdominal pain that presents to the ER. Children with constipation can have severe, sharp, and crampy abdominal pain. The pain typically comes and goes and can be located anywhere in the abdomen, although seems to be more commonly located on the left side. Children with constipation often have infrequent, large, or rock-hard stools. However, many children with constipation do not exhibit an obviously abnormal stooling pattern. I have cared for hundreds of patients with constipation that have a normal bowel movement (BM) daily. Upon performing an x-ray, a large amount of stool is found in the colon and their abdominal pain resolves after receiving an enema.

Children with constipation can have some vomiting, but it is uncommon to have repeated vomiting with this condition. If the vomit is green, the child may have an obstruction (a serious cause of bowel blockage). In this case, your child should be evaluated in an ER immediately.

Treatment of children with constipation can be difficult and requires heavy involvement from the parents. Children should eat a diet high in fiber (a lot of fruits and vegetables, but avoid bananas as they are constipating) and consume a lot of liquids (juice is great to help with constipation). Consuming large amounts of milk or cheese can also be constipating. Miralax® (Polyethylene Glycol) is an excellent over-the-counter medicine, which can help with constipation. It is a powder that is mixed with liquid (water, juice, etc.) and has no taste or bad odor. Often children with significant constipation may need more medication than just Miralax® to clean out their bowels. You should consult with your doctor regarding these cases. It is also important to train children to have a regular bowel movement schedule. This is only possible with children that are potty trained. After your child eats a meal, he/she should sit on the toilet and attempt to have a BM. Children should be encouraged to sit on the toilet even if they do not feel like they have to stool. This process, known as 'timed stooling,' will help regulate a child's body back to a normal pattern.

There are too many causes of abdominal pain to cover in this chapter. More important than knowing all of the causes of abdominal pain, it is key to understand symptoms that suggest serious causes of this type of pain. Abdominal pain that is severe, persistent, or localized (focused in one area), especially in the right lower side of the abdomen, is concerning. Children that have bloody or green vomit or bloody stools can have serious causes of their abdominal pain. Children with these symptoms should be evaluated by their doctor or seen in an ER immediately. Even if your child does not exhibit these symptoms, if you are concerned that your child has a serious abdominal condition, it is best to have him/her evaluated.

Key points to remember about
Abdominal Pain and Constipation:

*Serious causes of abdominal pain usually produce pain that is constant rather than intermittent.

*Have your child evaluated if you are concerned that there is a serious cause of the abdominal pain.

***Reasons to see your doctor**: If the pain is persistent or on the right lower side, there are signs of dehydration, or blood in the vomit or stool.

***Reasons to be seen in the ER**: If the pain is severe, there is severe dehydration, or your child vomits bile (green).

Chapter 9
Croup

Croup is a common condition that causes respiratory difficulty in the middle of the night. This condition is caused by a
virus that produces inflammation in the upper airway of children. This illness is one of the most common reasons that
parents bring their children to the ER for evaluation in the
middle of the night. In this chapter, I will discuss things you
can do to help your child at home and warnings signs that
signal the need to bring your child to the ER for evaluation.

Croup is typically a five-day illness that has the peak of
symptoms in the middle of that time frame. Children with
croup usually have a runny nose, congestion, and often have
fever. The hallmark symptom of croup is a barky cough,
which sounds like a seal barking. Children with croup have a
hoarse voice and cry. When the inflammation of croup becomes significant, children can have *stridor*, which is a high
pitched noise that is made upon inspiration (breathing in). As
with many respiratory illnesses, children with croup do not

usually eat well. It is most important to ensure that children drink sufficient amounts of liquid while sick.

As croup is caused by a virus, there is no cure for this illness (see *Chapter 10: Virus versus Bacteria*). However, there is a medicine that can be used to decrease the inflammation associated with croup. This medicine is a steroid medicine (Decadron®, which is also known as Dexamethasone), which is given in one or two doses depending upon the severity of the case. This short course of steroids is effective and safe and does not cause any of the side effects that are associated with the abuse of anabolic steroids. This treatment can lessen the severity of illness and shorten the course of the symptoms. There are other things that can mimic the symptoms of croup. Children that aspirate foreign bodies (e.g. a nut or coin, etc.) can sometimes have similar symptoms. Also, there are rare serious bacterial infections that can mimic the symptoms of croup. Your doctor will need to determine if any of these other conditions should be considered.

It is unclear why children with croup have more severe symptoms late at night or early in the morning, but it is definitely a fact. When children wake with a worsening cough and difficulty breathing (often the noisy breathing, *stridor*, mentioned earlier) it can be very alarming to parents. If your child has this particular difficulty breathing, there are a few easy home remedies that can help. First, take your child outside to breathe cold air. Parents often do not believe me because they believe that cold air is bad for an ill child. It is fine to bundle your child up when going outside to keep warm as it is the breathing of the cold air that is important. Many parents rush their child to the ER in the middle of the night due to this difficulty breathing. Upon arrival to the ER, the child is doing quite well and parents often try to convince the ER staff that the child was really sick at home. The explanation for this common occurrence is that children get to breathe cold air on the way to the ER and are significantly better upon arrival there. If the cold air does not stop the noisy breathing, take your child into the bathroom and start up a very hot shower. Do not put your child into the hot shower, but allow him/her to breathe the steamy air produced in the bathroom. If, after a few minutes of cool air and/or shower steam, your child is still having the noisy breathing, *stridor*, you should call your doctor or have your child seen in the ER.

There are several warning signs that should alert a parent that a child with croup should be evaluated by a doctor. If your child has respiratory difficulty (breathing fast, breathing hard, persistent noisy breathing) you should call your doctor or have your child evaluated in the ER. If your child has severe respiratory difficulty or is turning blue, call **911** to get immediate assistance. If your child is dehydrated, then see your doctor.

Key points to remember about Croup:

*There is no cure for croup, but a short course of steroids can help.

*If your child has noisy breathing, try having him/her breathe cool air and/or shower steam.

***Reasons to see your doctor**: If your child has respiratory difficulty (breathing fast, breathing hard, or persistent noisy breathing). If these symptoms occur at night when your doctor's office is closed, you should have your child evaluated in the ER.

***Reasons to be seen in the ER**: If your child has severe respiratory difficulty or is turning blue.

Chapter 10
Infections: Viruses versus Bacteria

There are two main types of infections that children acquire. The vast majority of these common infections are caused by viruses. A much smaller percentage of infections in children are caused by bacteria. A virus is a microscopic infectious agent that can cause many different symptoms depending upon the type of virus. Bacteria are also microscopic infectious agents, which can cause illness in children. The main difference between these types of infections is that antibiotics will work to cure bacterial infections, but will do nothing to help an infection caused by a virus. Most infections caused by viruses are less severe than bacterial infections.

The majority of illnesses that children acquire are caused by viruses. Common colds, croup, bronchiolitis, and vomiting and diarrhea (gastroenteritis) are all caused by viruses. Ear infections, pneumonia, and sinus infections are caused by bacteria and will likely require antibiotics. Your doctor should determine whether your child's symptoms are caused by a virus or a bacterium. You can discuss with your doctor why he/she has diagnosed the illness as a viral or bacterial infection.

Parents often want a prescription for antibiotics to help cure a child's illness. Even after I explain to parents that their child's symptoms are caused by a virus and that antibiotics will not help, I often receive pressure to prescribe an antibiotic. As a parent, I understand the desire to do anything you can to help your sick child. However, as a doctor, I understand the importance of only prescribing antibiotics when indicated. Parents often tell me that the last time their child had respiratory symptoms, he/she received a course of antibiotics that resolved the symptoms in a few days. I believe that their child's symptoms would have likely resolved on their own if antibiotics had not been prescribed. The improper use of antibiotics (i.e. using antibiotics for a viral infection) leads to the growing problem of antibiotic resistance.

Antibiotic resistance is the ability of bacteria to withstand the effects of antibiotics. This happens when bacteria in your body mutate so that antibiotics are no longer effective to fight that bacteria. This process of resistance occurs by the repeated exposure to the same antibiotic. It can also occur when the bacteria are not completely killed, as can happen when people do not take the full course of antibiotics prescribed. These bacteria grow and develop the ability to resist antibiotics. This, unfortunately, has become a common and increasing problem in medicine. Due to this resistance, many antibiotics do not work for certain types of infections. Remember that pressuring your doctor into prescribing antibiotics may actually cause more harm than good for your child.

There are a few viruses that can be treated with medications. These medications, called antivirals, are targeted to specifically fight a particular virus. The most common of these medicines can be used to treat Herpes infections. Another common antiviral can be used to treat Influenza infections (see *Chapter 11: Influenza*). You will need to discuss with your doctor if one of these medications would be indicated to help your child.

Key points to remember about Viral versus Bacterial Infections:

*Very few viruses can be treated with medications.

*Using antibiotics to treat a virus will not cure the symptoms, but can cause antibiotic resistance.

*Discuss with your doctor why he/she has diagnosed the illness as a viral or bacterial infection.

*Discuss with your doctor whether or not antibiotics are indicated in your child's illness.

*Do not pressure your doctor into prescribing antibiotics if he/she believes that your child has a virus.

Chapter 11
Influenza

Influenza and the Swine Flu (H1N1) are both viruses. The Influenza virus has two main types, A and B. There are many subtypes within the A and B groupings. The H1N1 Swine Flu virus is one of the types of Influenza A. In this chapter, I will discuss how to care for a child with an Influenza infection and what warning signs need to be monitored.

Influenza is a common virus that affects individuals each winter. With Influenza, there are certain age groups that are considered as high risk for serious complications. The high risk age groups include people over 65 years, children under five years, people with chronic medical problems (e.g. significant asthma, heart disease, diabetes, kidney disease, neurological diseases, etc.), and pregnant women. Each year in the United States, Influenza kills between 30,000 and 40,000 people. About five times this number (approximately 200,000 people) are hospitalized annually due to complications of

Influenza. The majority of these deaths and hospitalizations occur in people over the age of 65.

The spread of Influenza occurs through respiratory secretions. This happens when people cough and sneeze and spread the disease to another. It is also possible to touch something that has the Influenza virus on it and then become infected by touching your hand with the virus to your nose or mouth. Examples of this include handrails, elevator buttons, grocery carts, etc.

Several preventative methods can help thwart the spread of respiratory illnesses such as Influenza. These measures include washing your hands frequently, covering your nose/mouth when sneezing/coughing, and avoiding contact with people who are ill. Also, there is a vaccine against Influenza. As a doctor, I believe in the vaccine and have recommended it to the children who I care for. Additionally, an even stronger endorsement in favor of the vaccine is that my wife, children, and I are vaccinated against Influenza each year.

The symptoms of Influenza are fever, chills, cough, body aches, sore throat, runny nose, and headaches. Some people also have vomiting and diarrhea with Influenza infections. The concerning signs to watch for in children include: difficulty breathing, breathing fast, lethargy (so sleepy that your child is nearly unarousable), dehydration (see *Chapter 2: Vomiting, Diarrhea, and Dehydration*), excessive irritability (will not console even if being held), and turning blue. If your child is breathing fast or is dehydrated, you should have him/her evaluated by your doctor. If your child is lethargic, irritable, has severe respiratory distress, or turns blue, you should have him/her seen in the ER.

How can you help a child with Influenza? Treat the fever with Ibuprofen and Acetaminophen (see *Chapter 1: Fever*). There are medicines that can treat Influenza if it is caught early enough. These medicines are typically only effective if started within 48 hours of the onset of illness. Discuss with your doctor whether or not these medicines would be appropriate for your child. It is also important to ensure that your child stays hydrated. Constantly encourage your children to drink (more than to eat) while they are sick.

Key points to remember about Influenza:

*Encourage your child to drink enough to stay well hydrated.
*Wash hands, cover your nose/mouth when sneezing/coughing, and avoid contact with people who are ill to prevent the spread of Influenza.

***Reasons to see your doctor**: Your child has difficulty breathing or is dehydrated.

***Reasons to be seen in the ER**: Your child has severe respiratory distress, turns blue, is lethargic, or irritable.